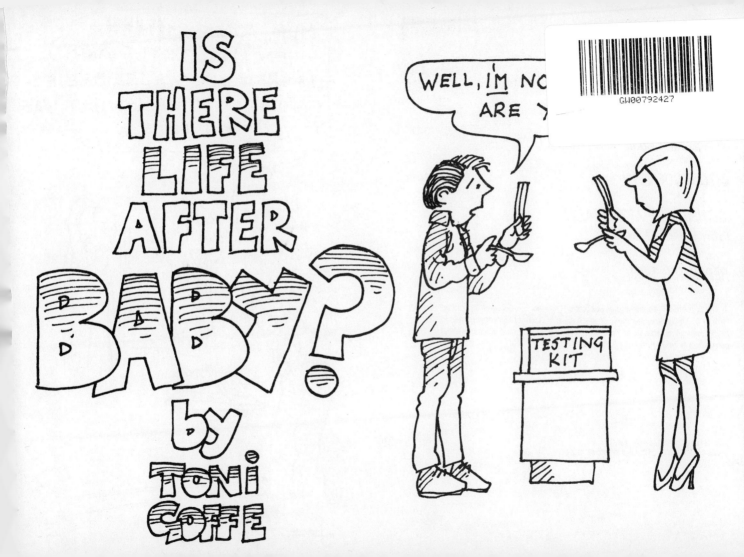

First published in Great Britain by
Pendulum Gallery Press
56 Ackender Road, Alton, Hants GU34 1JS

© TONI GOFFE 1993

IS THERE LIFE AFTER BABY?
ISBN 0-948912-23-5

REPRINTED 1993

PRINTED IN GREAT BRITAIN BY
UNWIN BROTHERS LTD, OLD WOKING, SURREY

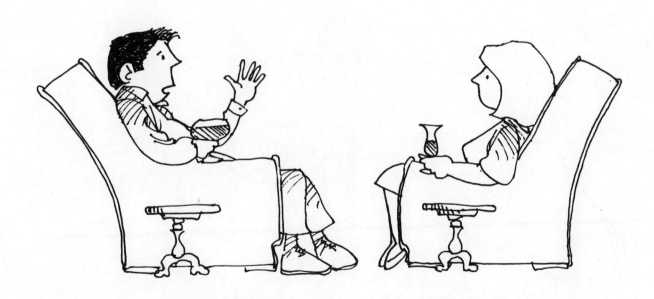

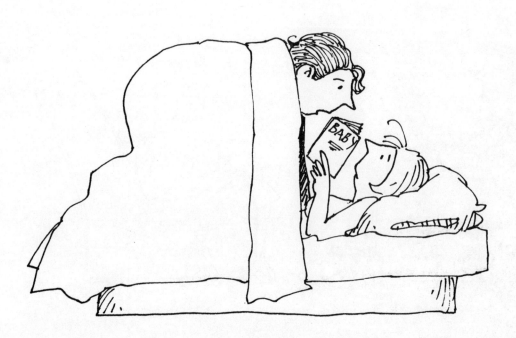

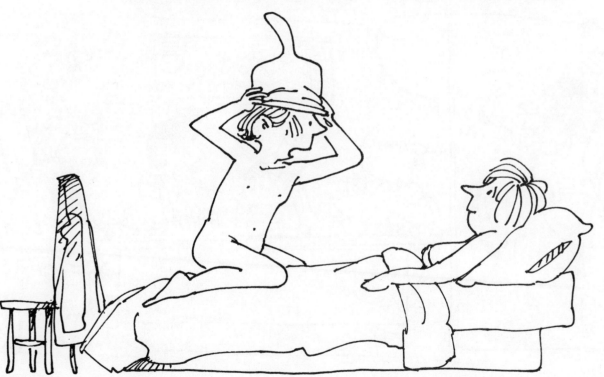

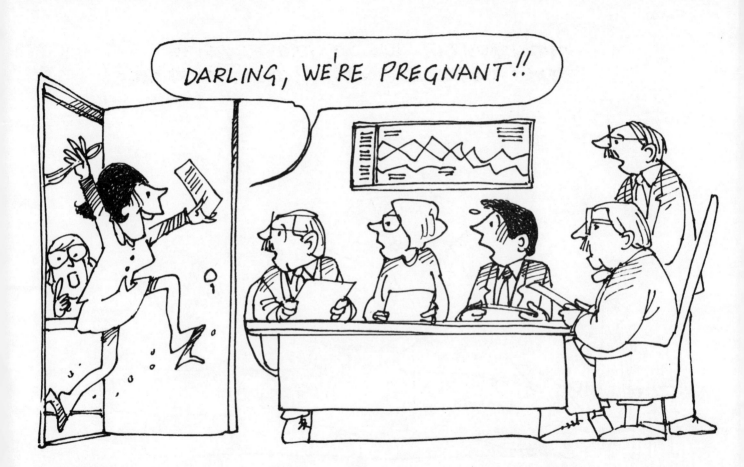

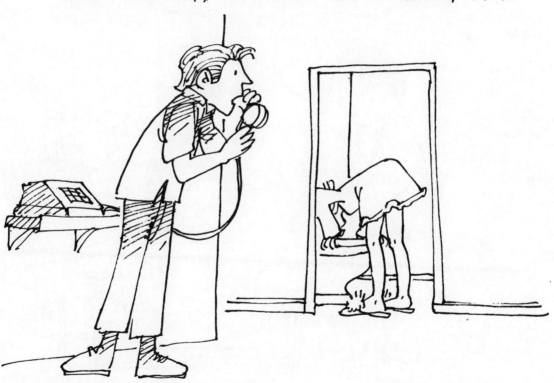

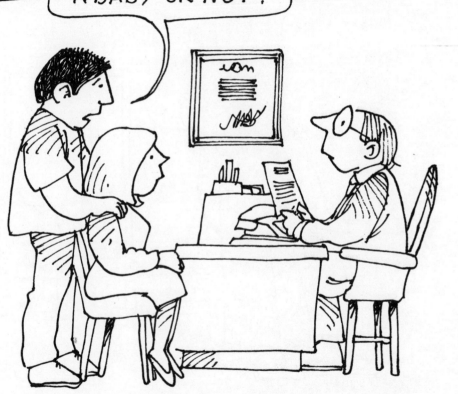

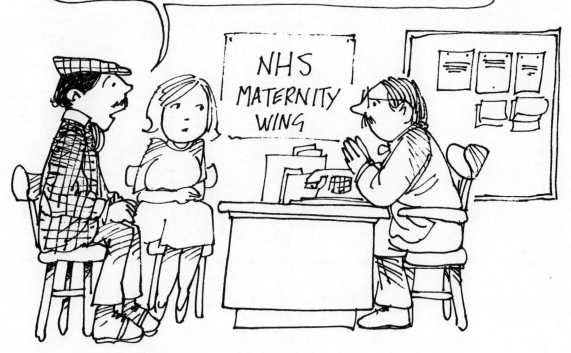

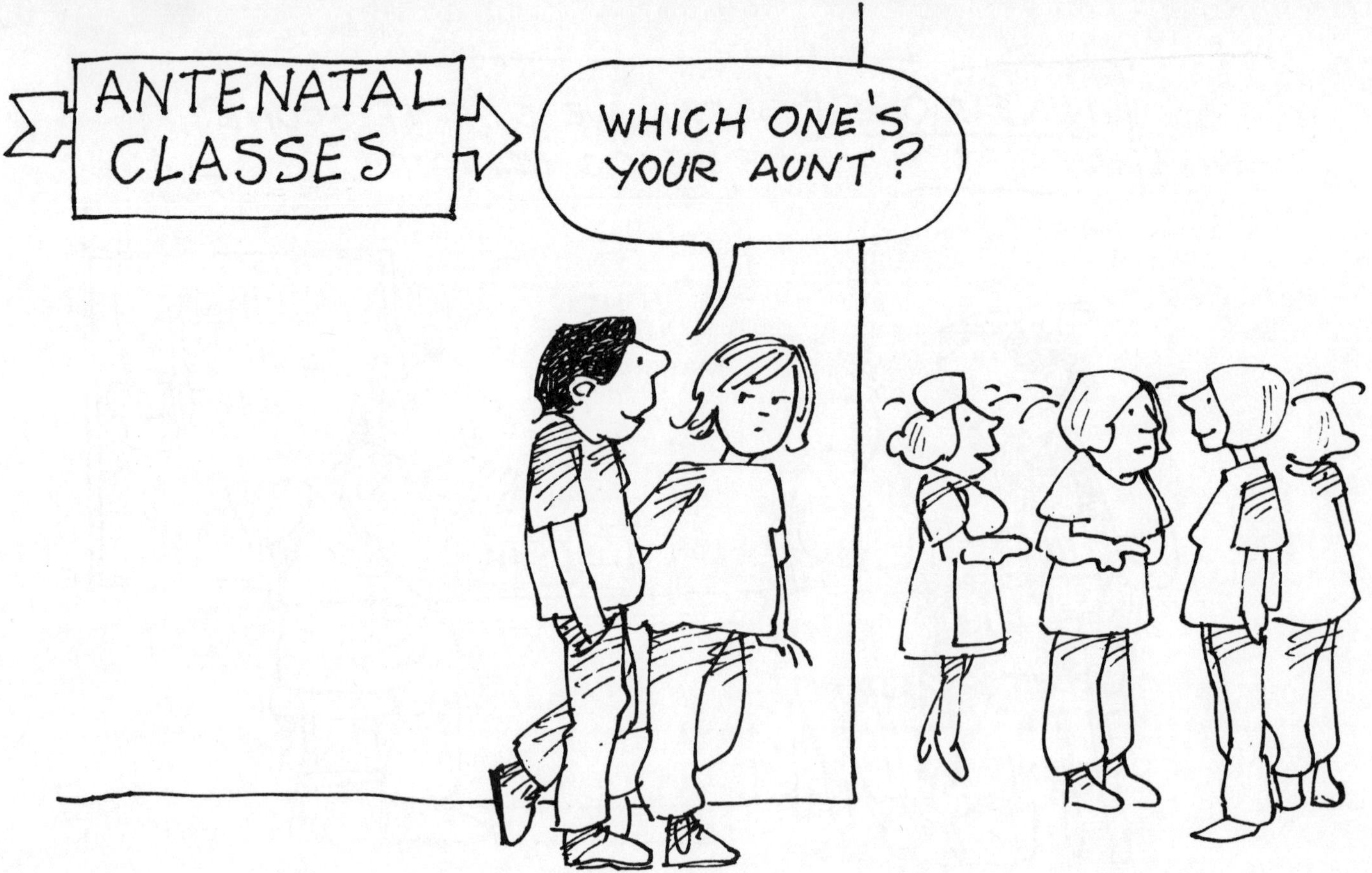
ANTENATAL CLASSES
WHICH ONE'S YOUR AUNT?

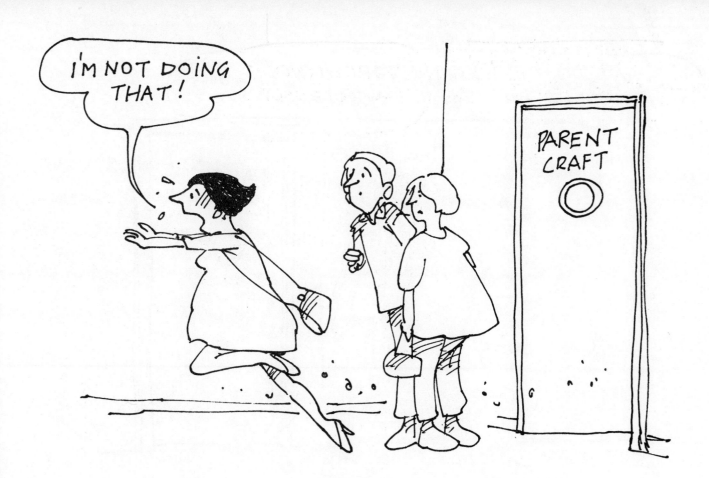

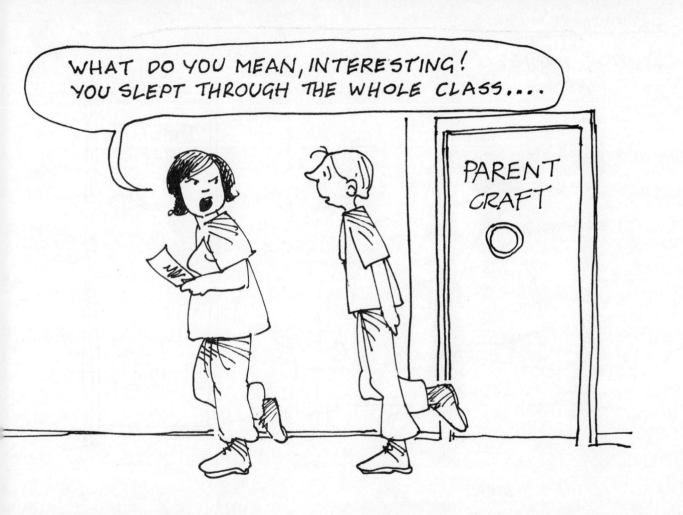

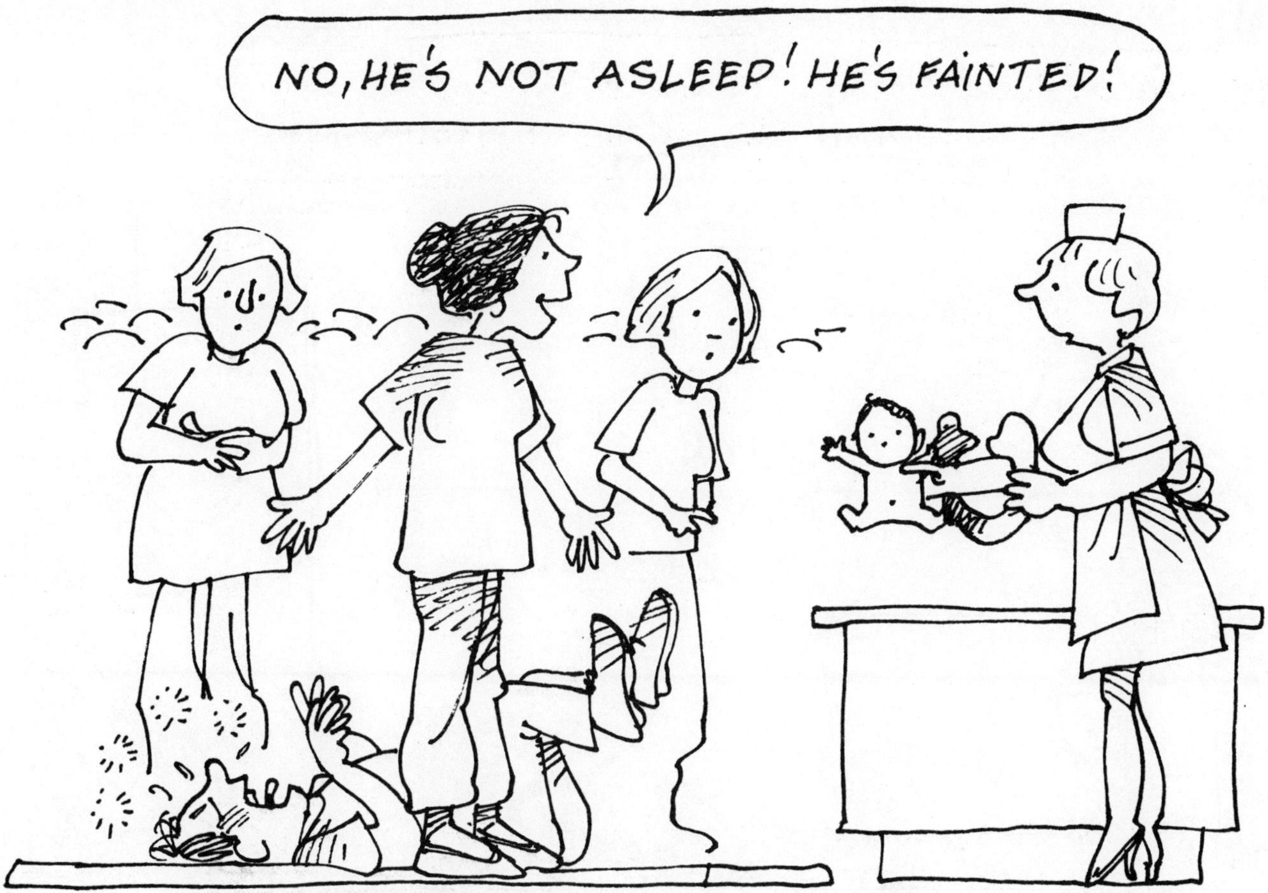
NO, HE'S NOT ASLEEP! HE'S FAINTED!

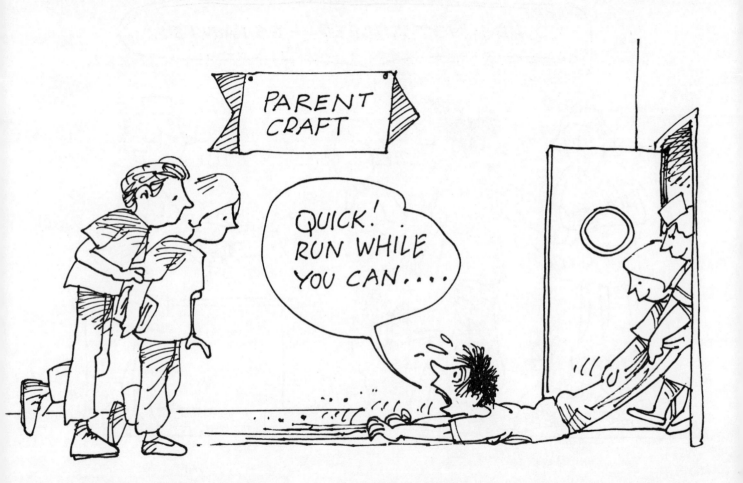

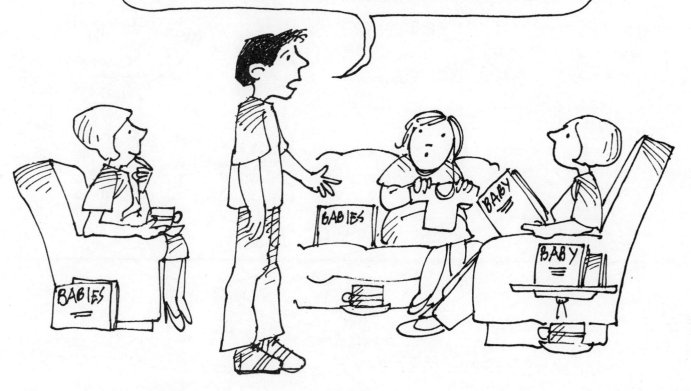

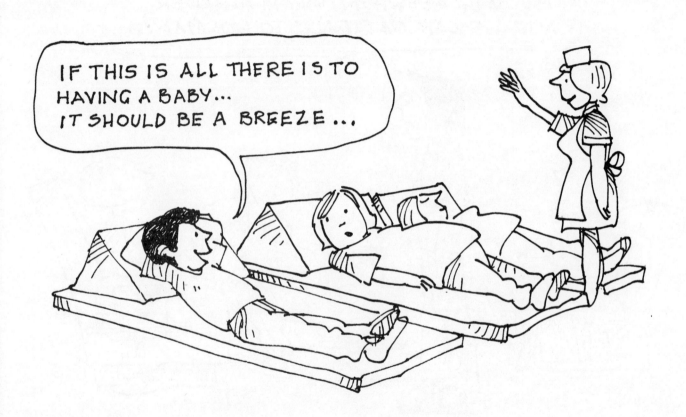

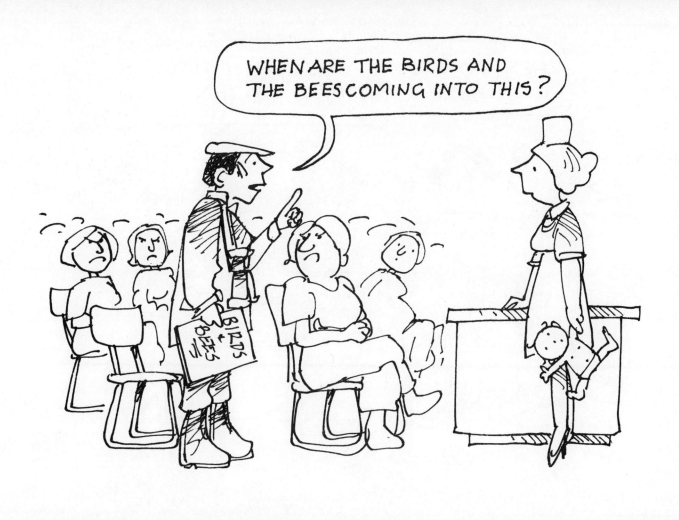

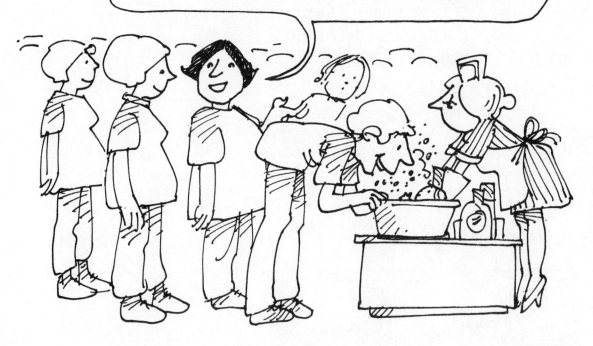

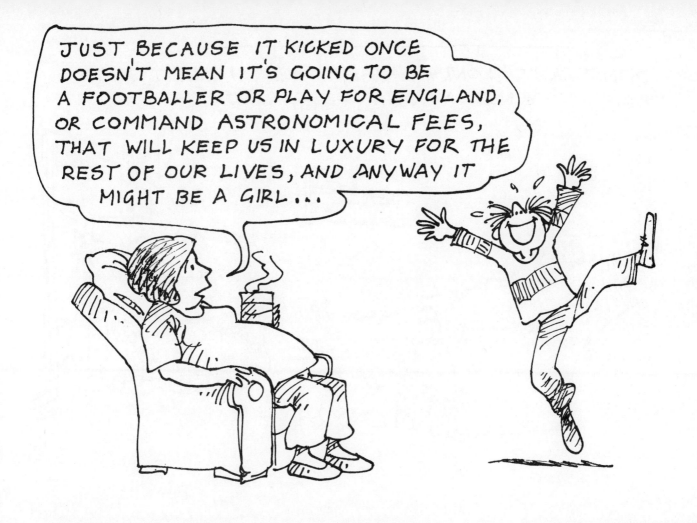

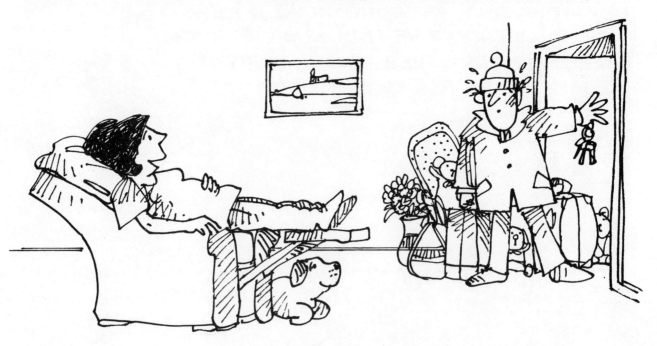

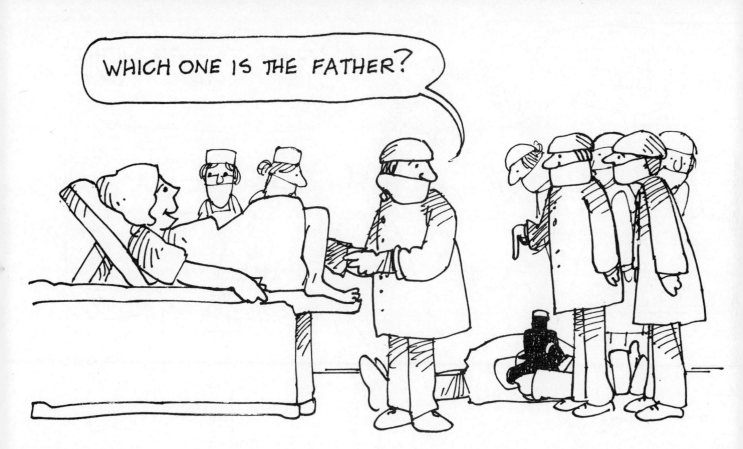

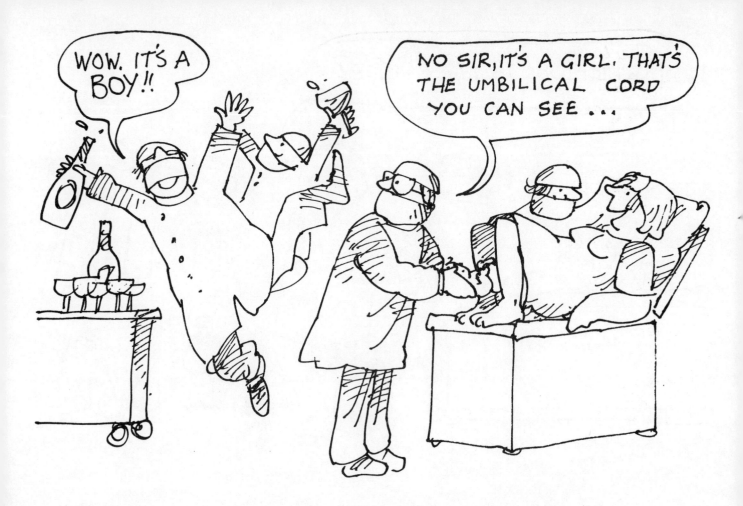

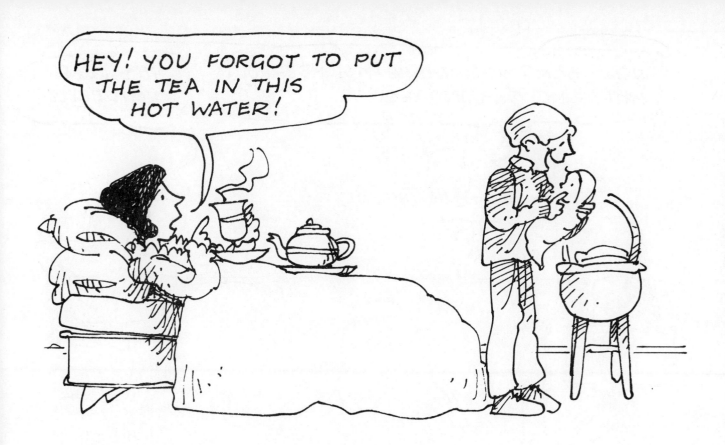

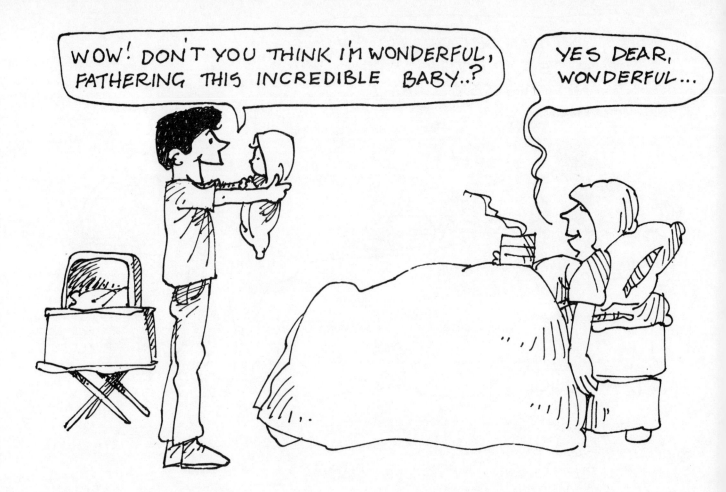

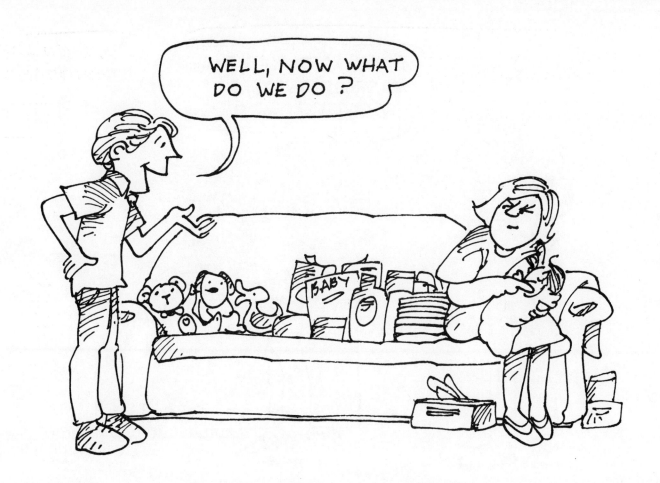

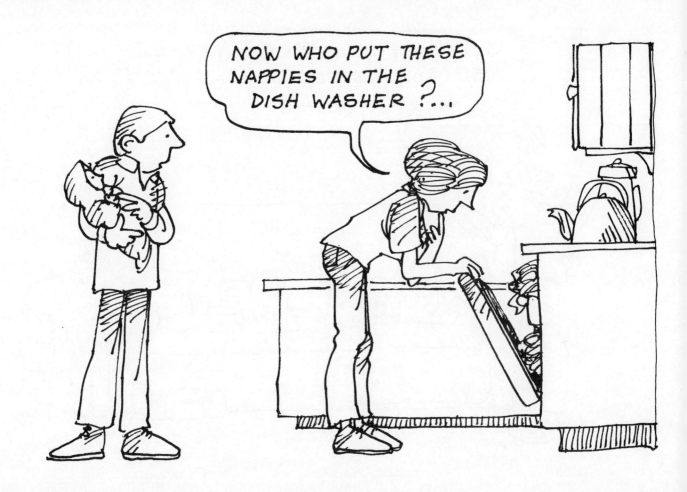

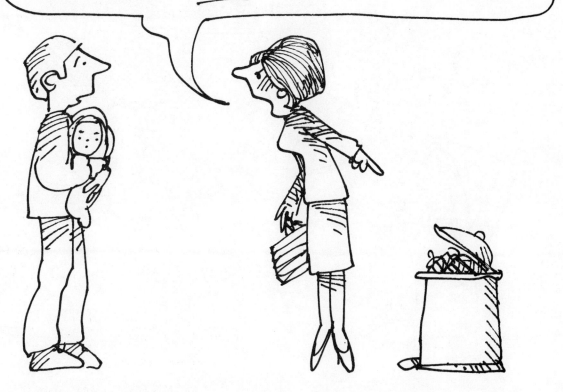

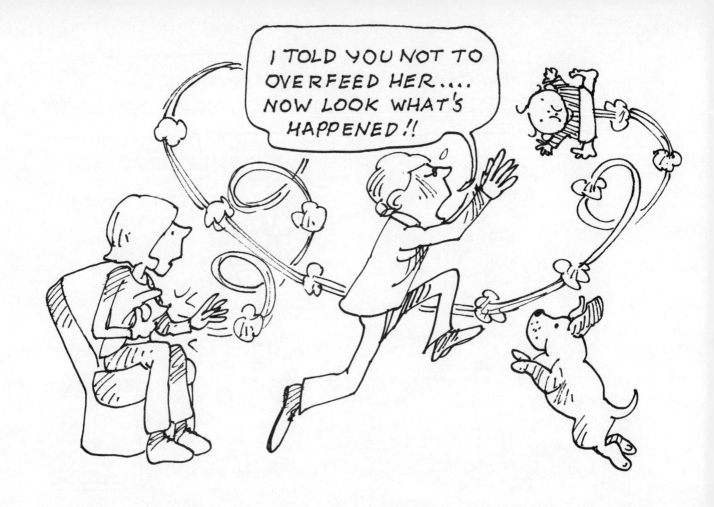

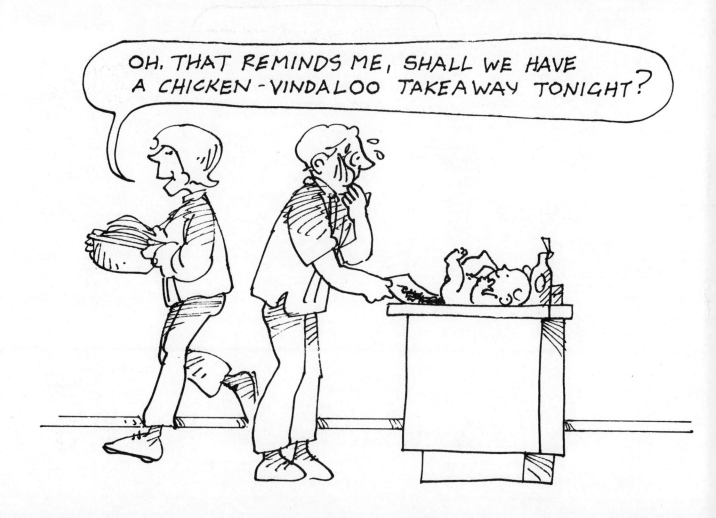

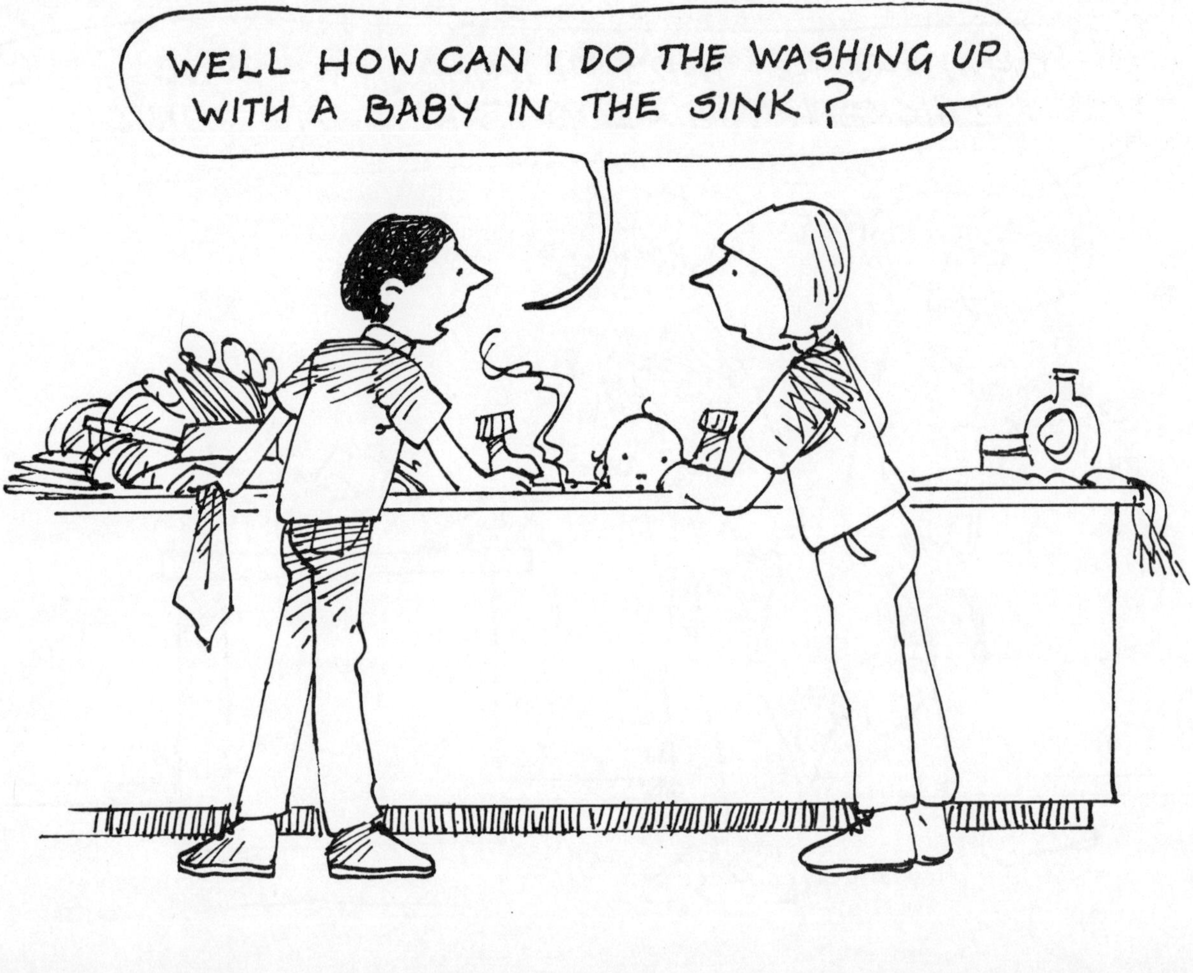
WELL HOW CAN I DO THE WASHING UP WITH A BABY IN THE SINK?

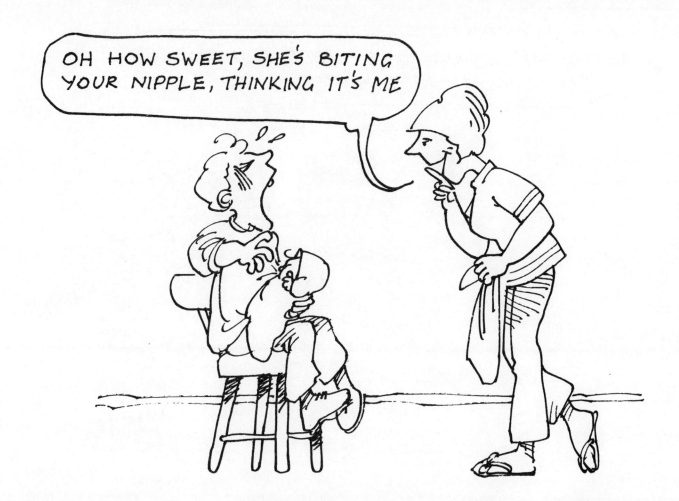

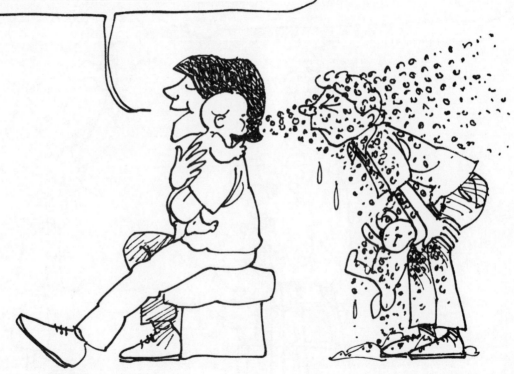

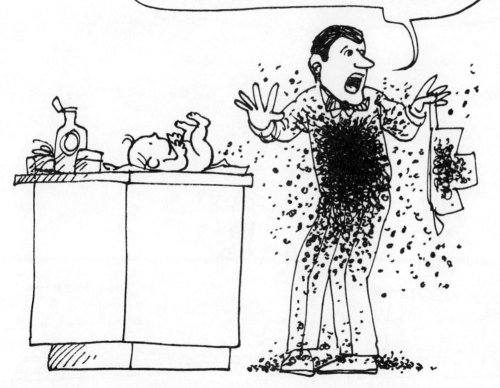
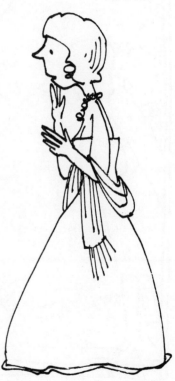

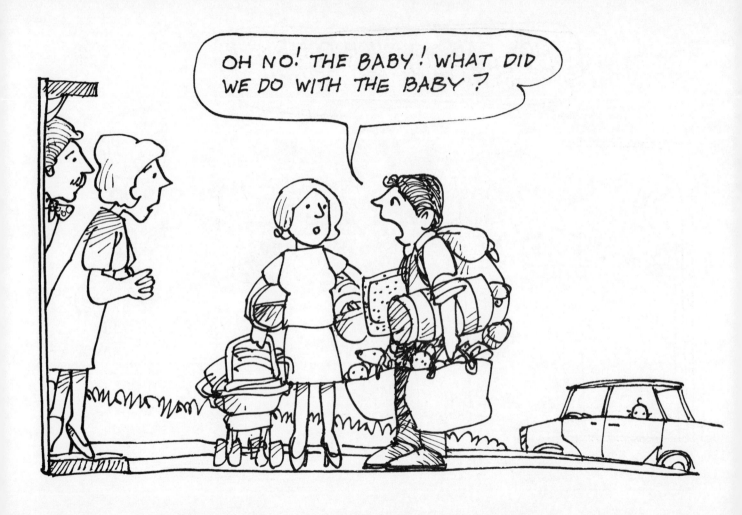

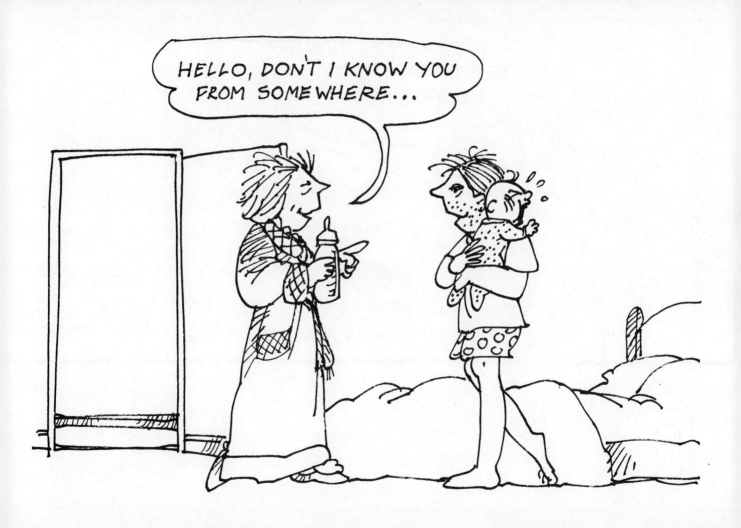

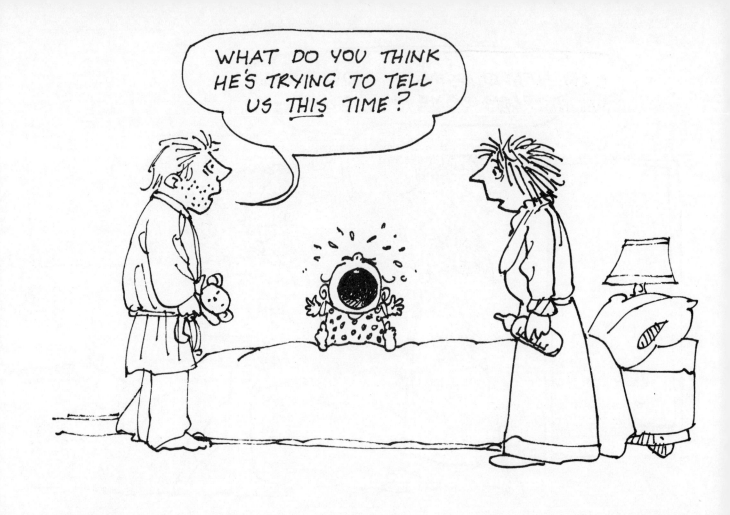

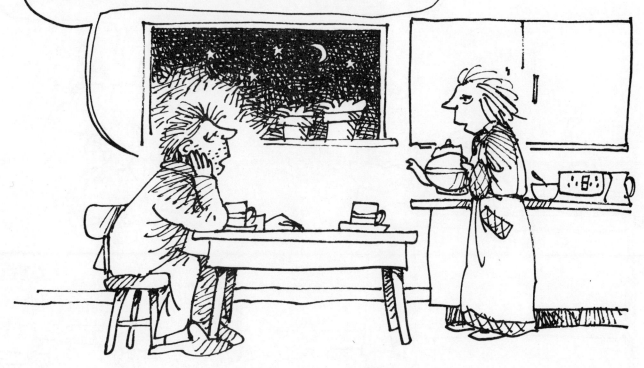

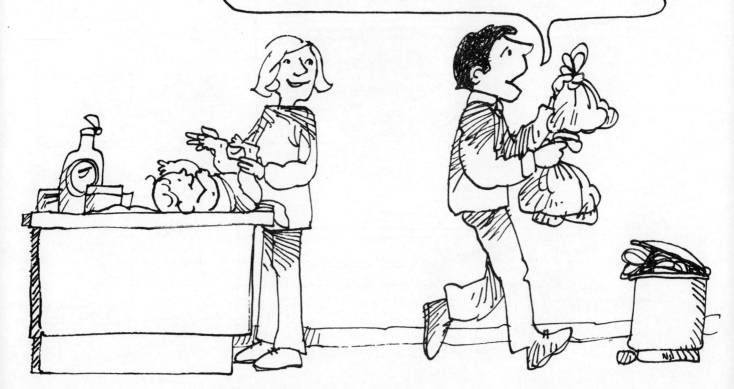

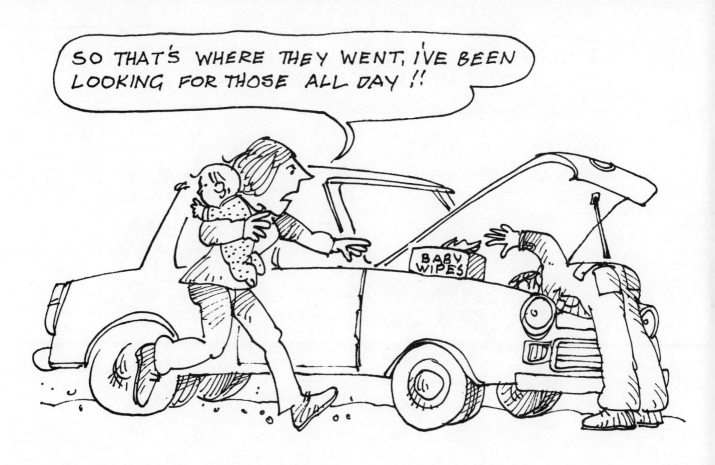

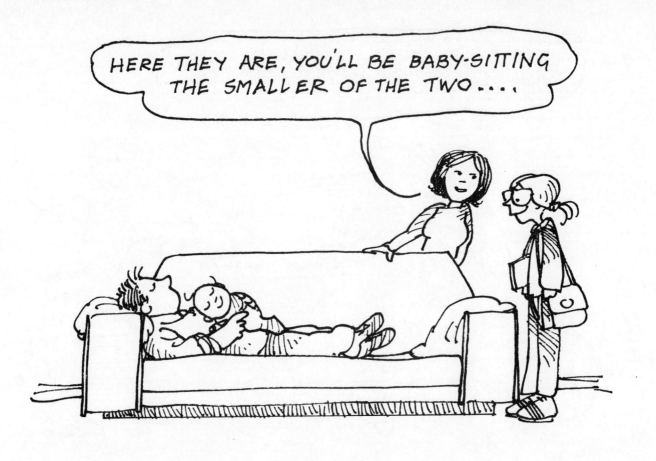

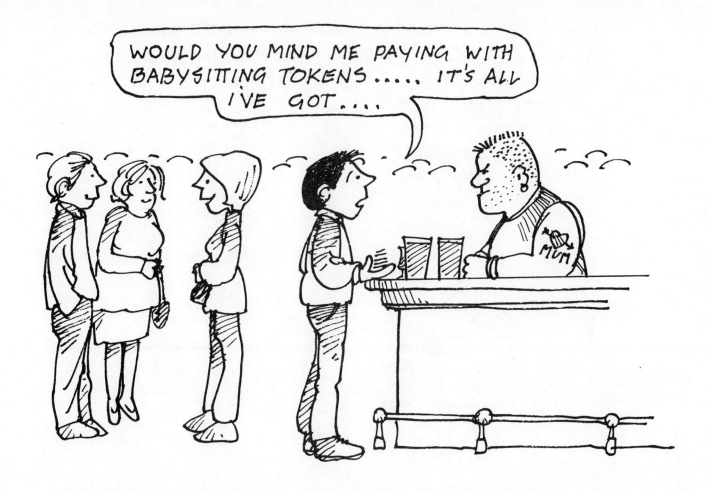

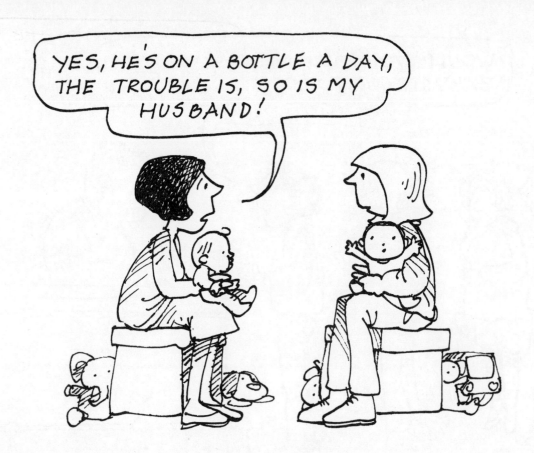

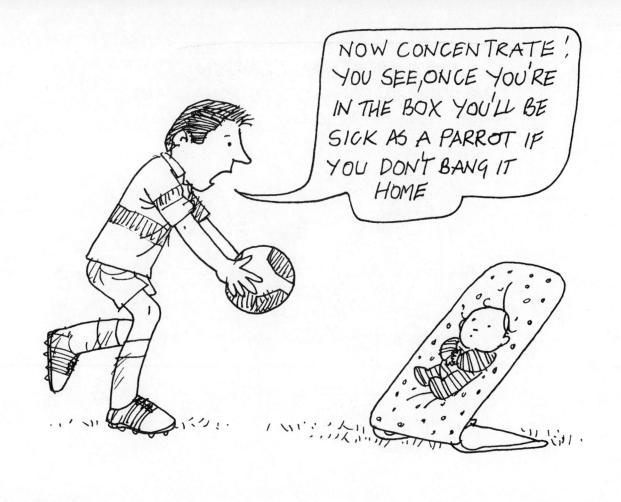

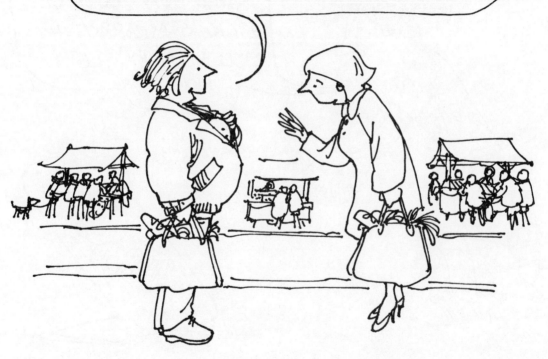

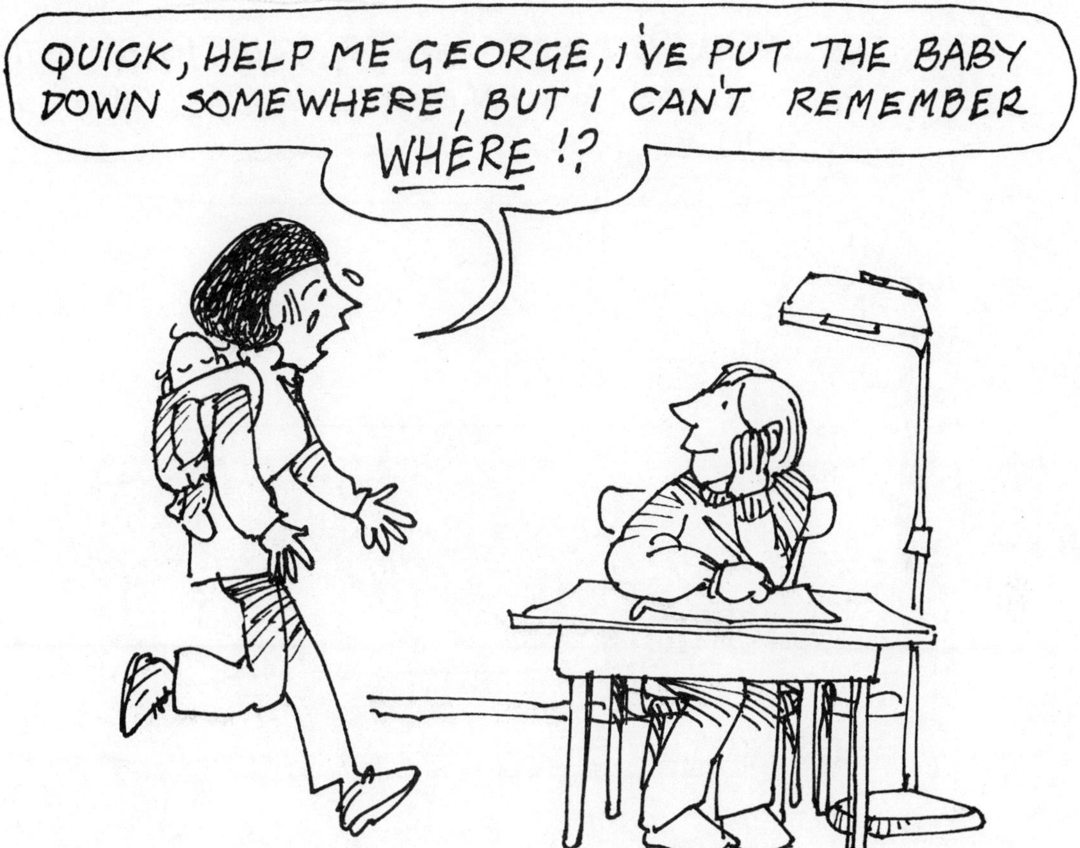
QUICK, HELP ME GEORGE, I'VE PUT THE BABY DOWN SOMEWHERE, BUT I CAN'T REMEMBER WHERE !?

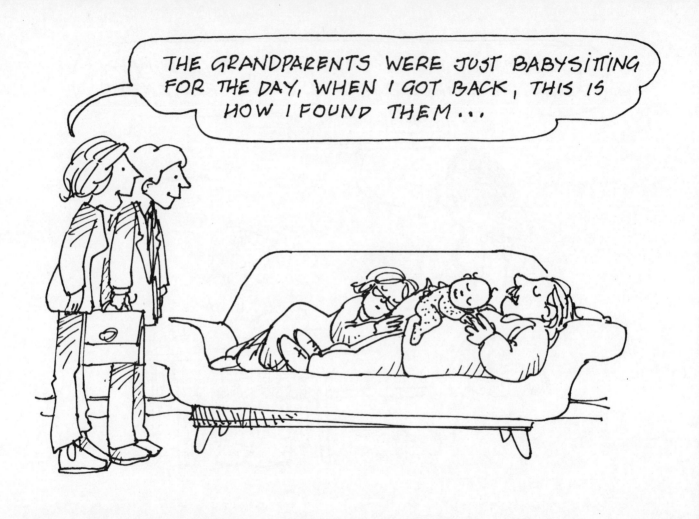

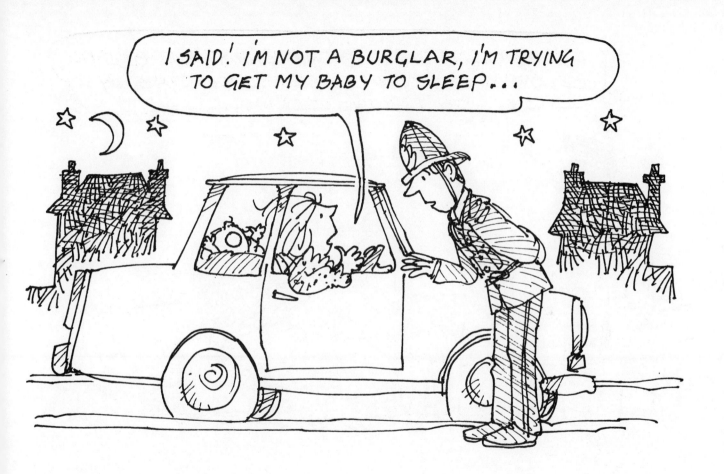

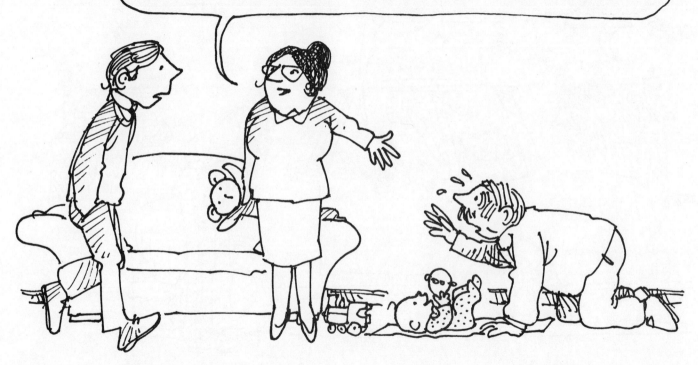

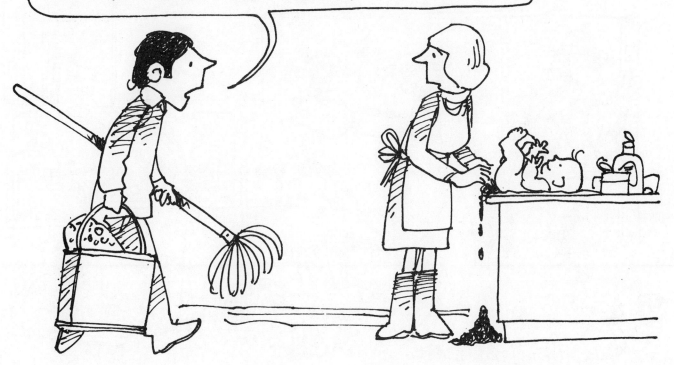

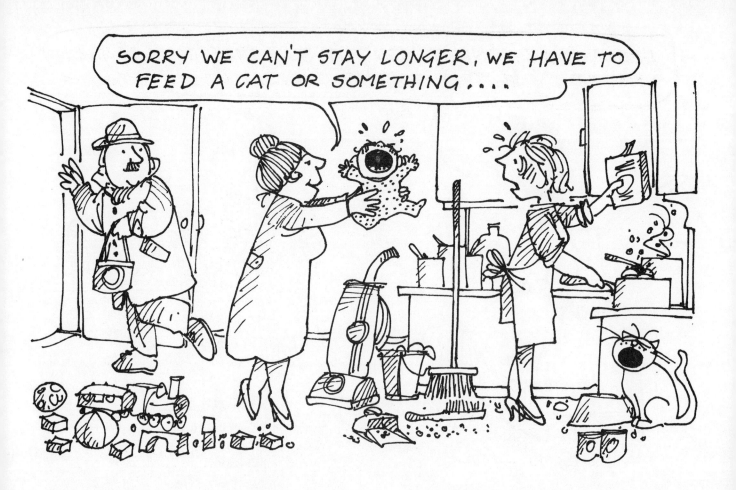

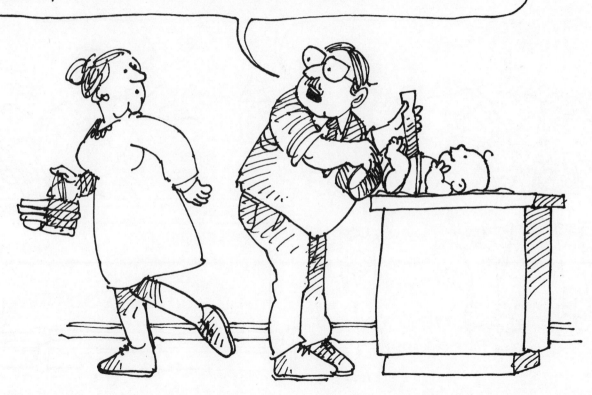

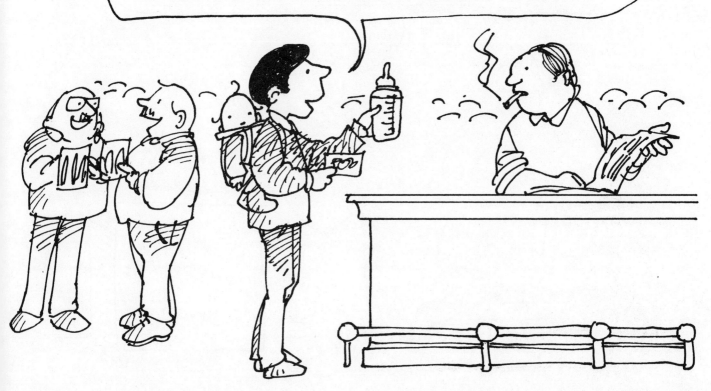

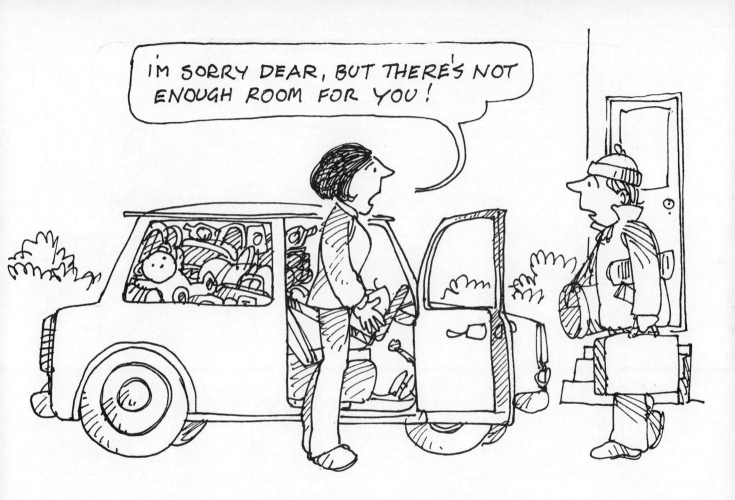

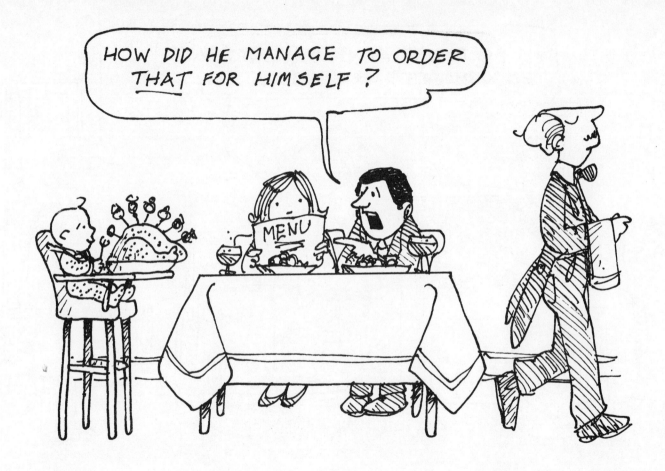

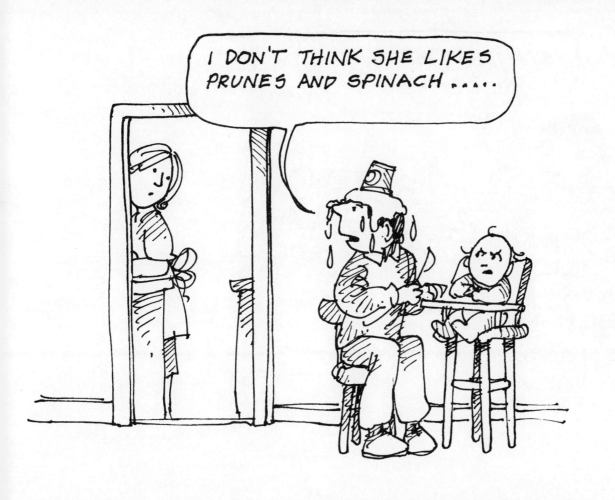

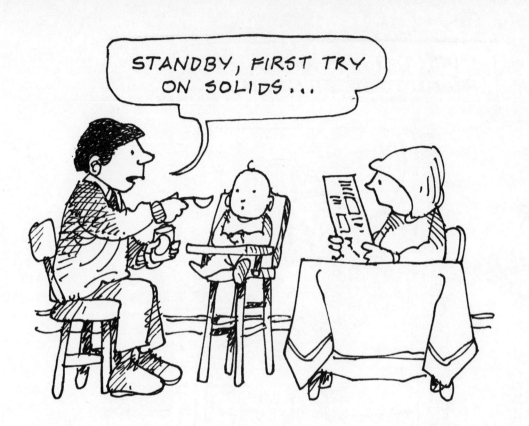

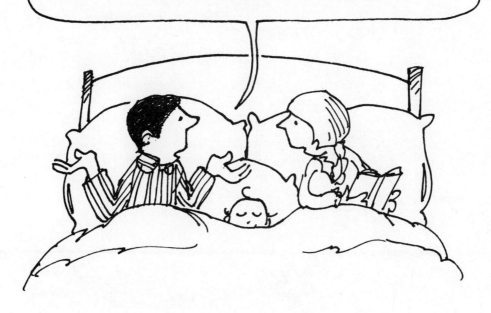

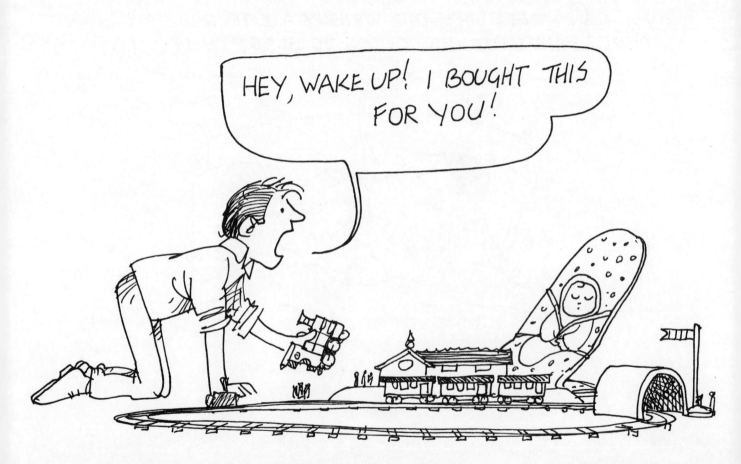

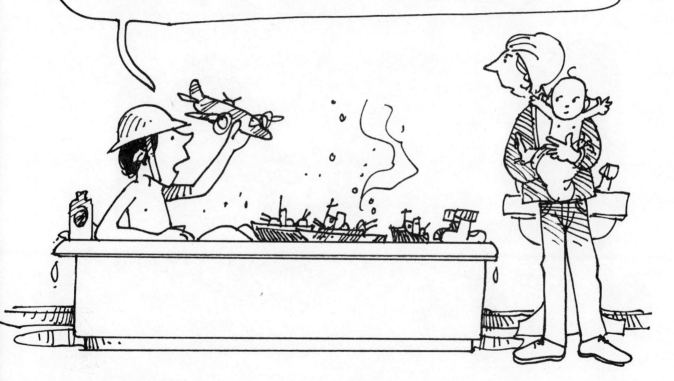

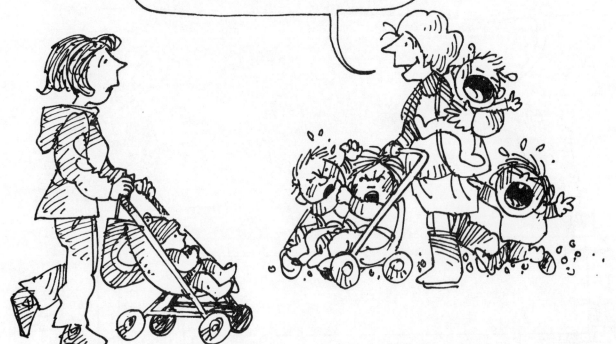

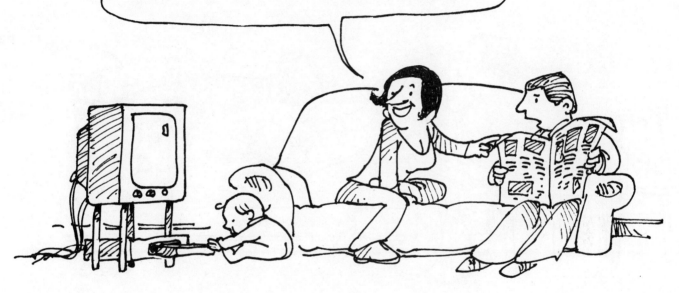

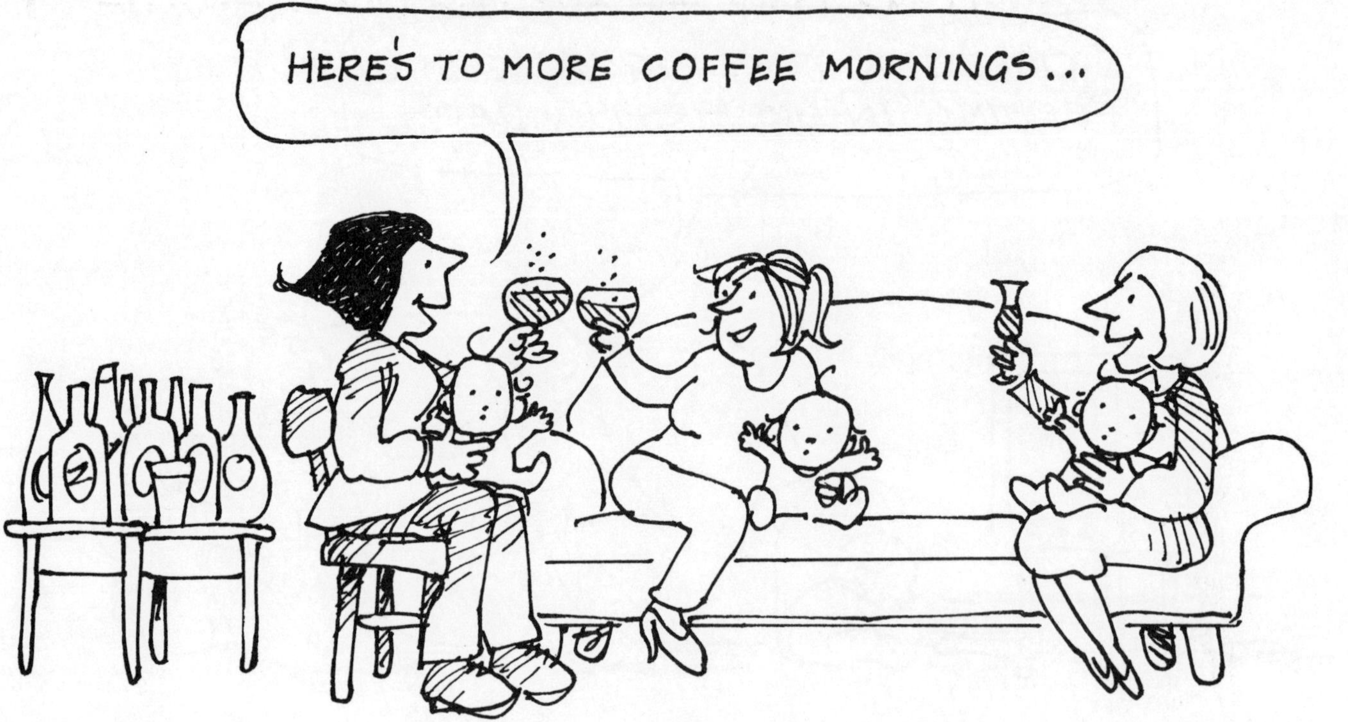
HERE'S TO MORE COFFEE MORNINGS...

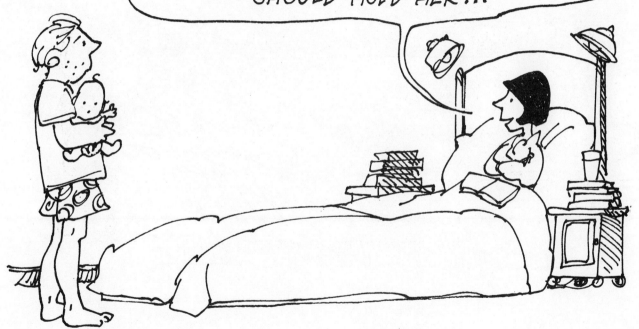

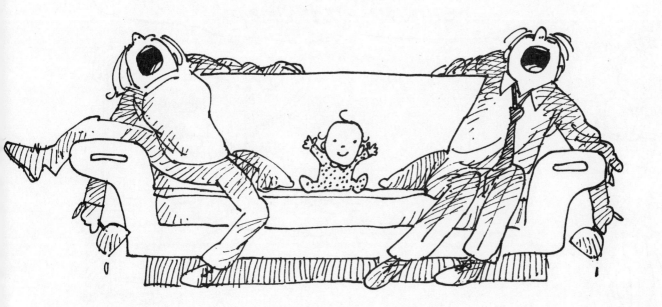